Poems from a Purposeful Life

POEMS FROM A PURPOSEFUL LIFE

Published by: MAVEN Project PO Box 156781
San Francisco, California 94115
https://www.mavenproject.org/

Editors: Barbara Loeb, MD, LoAn Nguyen, MD & Jill Einstein, MD
Cover Art: Tom E. Norris, MD

Printed in the United States of America

ISBN - 979-8-9869154-4-9

Poems from a Purposeful Life

By Tom E. Norris, MD

Edited by: Barbara Loeb, MD,
LoAn Nguyen, MD & Jill Einstein, MD

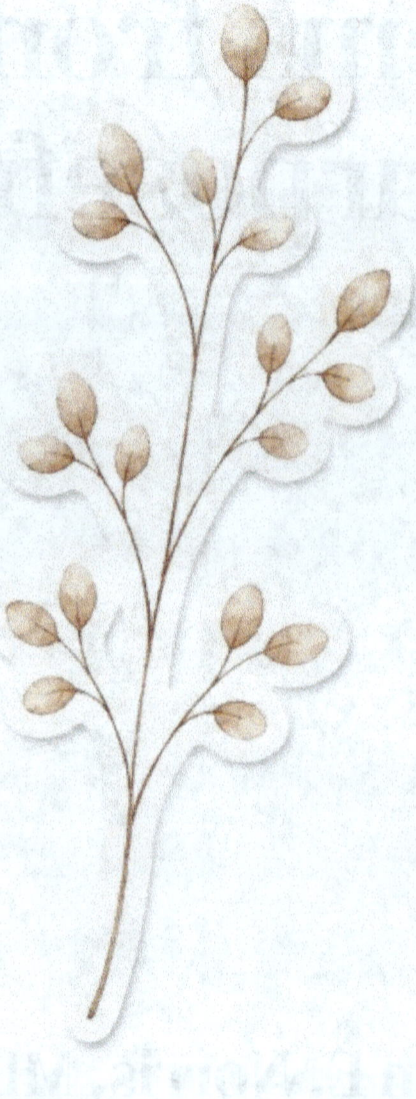

Dedicated to

Sandy Norris
My lifelong partner

Table of Contents

Forward **1**

Preface **3**

I Must Do. . . Purpose 5

Early On **7**

Childhood Memories Sixty Years On 3

Tom: A Name 4

ReNew 6

Discovering I Need Nature 8

Orange 10

Haikus 12

Pandemic & Volunteering **15**

The Irony of Joy in a Pandemic 17

COVID: A Travel Companion 18

A Place to Belong 20

Thanks! 22

Reflections on Aging 24

Be One with the World 26

Looking Deeper **29**

Tunnel Vision 30

A Physical Hole or an Emotional Depression? 32

Inside the Chest 34

Beyond the Surface 36
Helping a Dying Patient 38
Remembrance 41
Choices 42
Thoughts on Renewal 44

Life Journey **47**

Sum of My Bookshelf 48
If I Could Only Share What I Know Now 50
Thinking or Feeling 52
Thoughts on Unconditional Love 54
Querencia 56
Time to Sell the Boat 58
Just Like That! 60
Reflections on the End of Life 62
Hope 64
Skagit Tulips 67
Hill 68

Epilogue - Capstone **70**

Acknowledgements **72**

About the Author **74**

Table of Images

Photos and Wood Crafting by Tom E. Norris

Cover: San Juan Sunset

Wave Bowl in Walnut

Three Bowls on Black Surface

Natural Edge Spalted Maple Bowl

Maple Bowl

Filigreed Maple Bowl

Three Maple Bowls

Grooved Maple Bowl

Skagit Tulips in Tom's Garden

Forward

I met Tom Norris in 2016 when we were both doing Physician Leadership Coaching for Studer Group. At that time, I knew nothing about his way with words and talent for transforming a simple word prompt within 10 minutes into a clever and meaningful verse. Beyond this I was unaware of the elegant bowls he crafted out of maple and walnut.

We reconnected in 2021 when we both volunteered as mentors for MAVEN Project, a national nonprofit organization working to address the social, racial, and economic inequities in health care.

In response to the pandemic and their transitions to retirement, Tom along with other MAVEN Project physician volunteers, formed a reflective writing community called "Narrative and Humanity." In 2022 after meeting monthly for a year, the group published their writing and artwork into a collection, *Reflections on Medicine and Humanity* and then in 2024, a second book, *Medicine and Humanity: Narratives of Many Colors.*

Due to his ability to create poetry in an amazing way, Tom became known as our poet laureate. His contributions were always profound and inspiring.

In this volume, *Poems from a Purposeful Life*, we are honored to share Tom's poetic offerings along with photos of his woodworking objects. I have had the privilege to enjoy these works, and I know you will as well.

Barbara Loeb, MD, editor

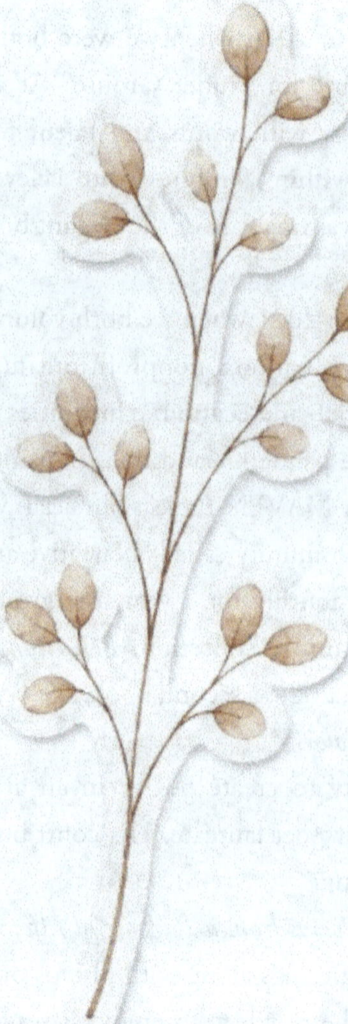

Preface

I retired from academic family medicine at the University of Washington in 2016. I had been a very busy family doctor, in multiple settings, since completing my residency in 1976. After spending three years as a consultant, I completely retired.

Upon full retirement, I sought volunteer opportunities to give me a chance to contribute and to provide me with a sense of purpose. One of my friends worked at a Federally Qualified Community Health Center (FQHC) and was exposed to MAVEN Project. I investigated the program and was very pleased with the opportunities it offered for mentoring and consulting in support of FQHC's.

Little did I know that there was much more to MAVEN than just its prime function. I soon discovered MAVEN Project's "Narrative and Humanity" writing group. This amazing group of retired doctors who volunteer with MAVEN, meet monthly and write together, in response to a specific prompt.

I have been writing poetry for most of my life, and this group has given me an unprecedented chance to write poems and share them with others. Most of the poems in this volume were written as part of this unique experience.

Tom E. Norris, MD, author

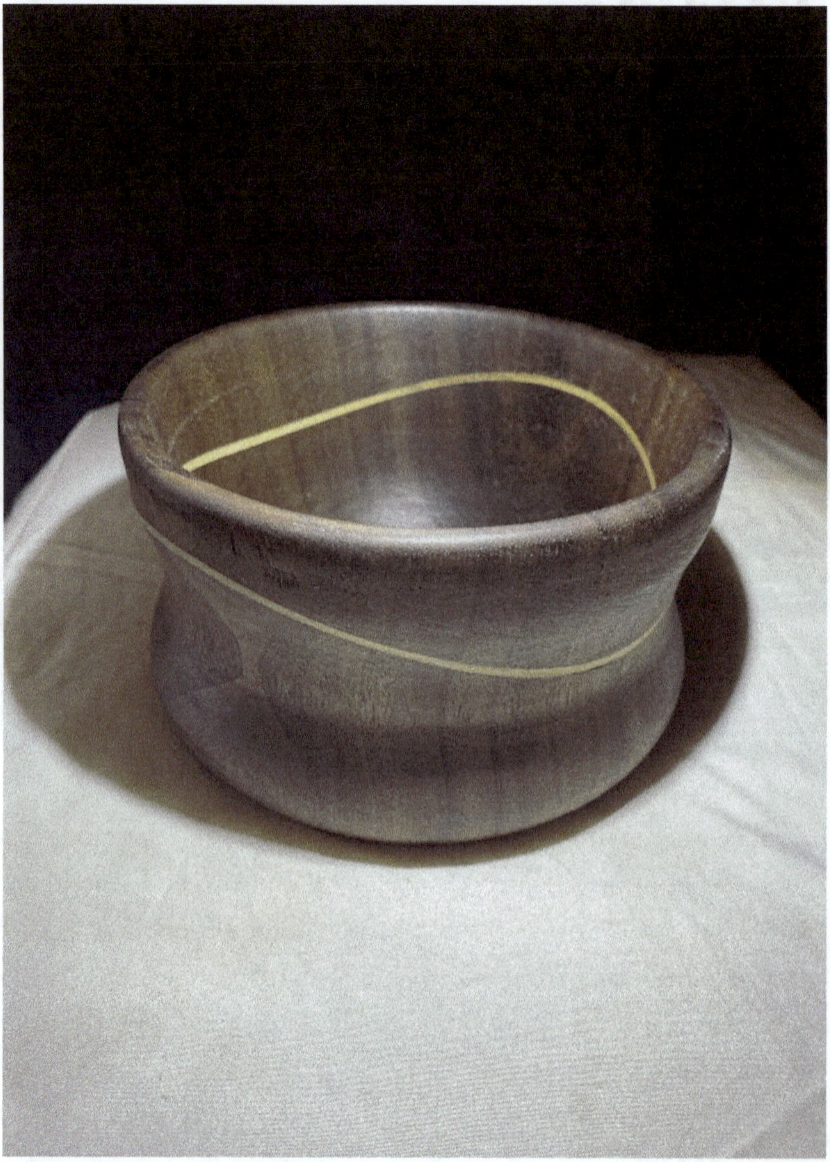

Wave Bowl in Walnut

I Must Do. . . Purpose

I must live a life filled with purpose.
There must be a reason to go.
This gives a clear path through the circus.
It tells me the course I must row!

For life with no purpose is madness,
A strange and bewildering place.
It is full of disorder and sadness—
And lacking of joy and of grace.

So, purpose is something well-needed,
For a life full and complete and sublime.
It's just like a garden fresh weeded--
And it's what can keep us in our prime.

Early On

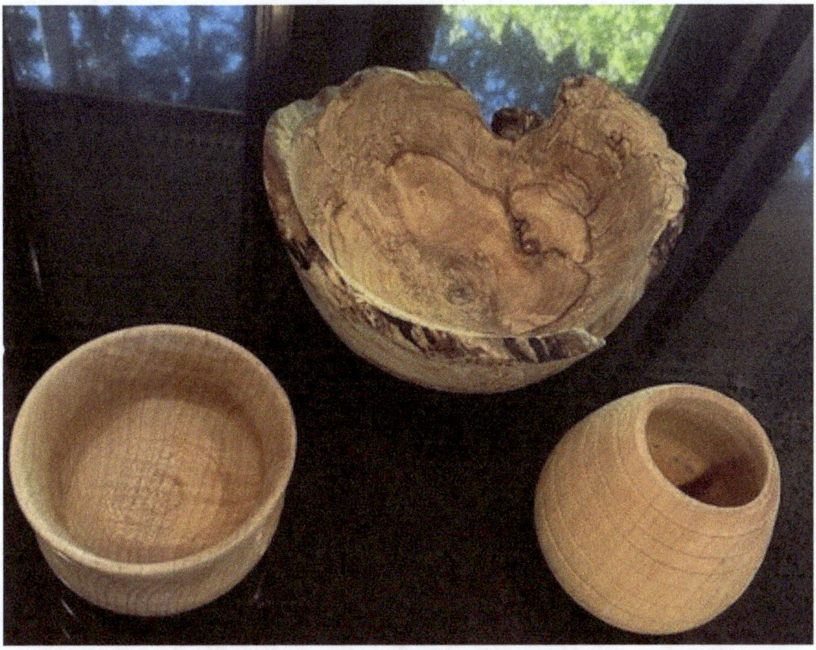

Three Bowls on Black Surface

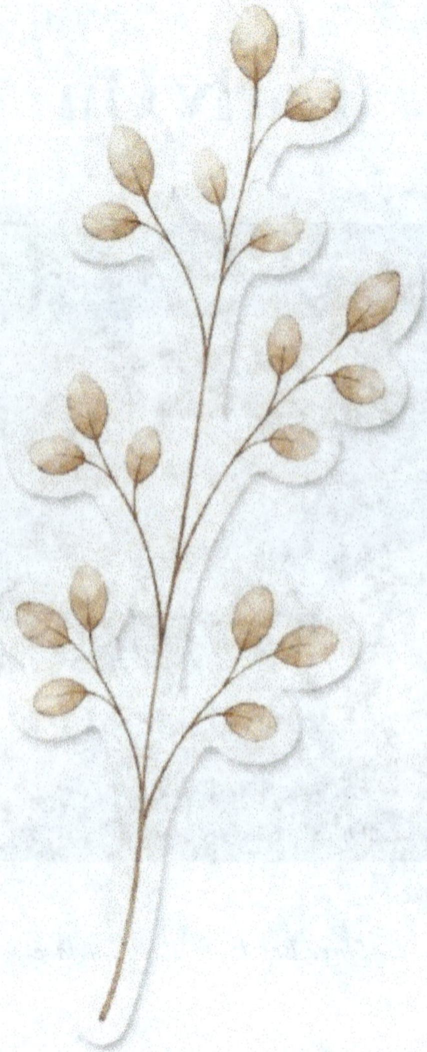

Childhood Memories Sixty Years On

Childhood memories do not flow,
From start to end, like video.
Instead, snapshots, a slice of life.
Some happy, some sad, some filled with strife.

As the years pile up from here to there.
I grow older, wiser, lose my hair.
Instead of focus, crystal clear.
Now edges fuzz, the scenes do blear.

From sequences, all lined up and straight.
To random pictures, through the gate.
From sharp edged photos every day,
To fuzz soft scenes, like by Monet.

Let's keep the happy and the good.
The smiles from our old neighborhood.
Let's lose the pain, the strife, the fear.
So childhood memories improve each year.

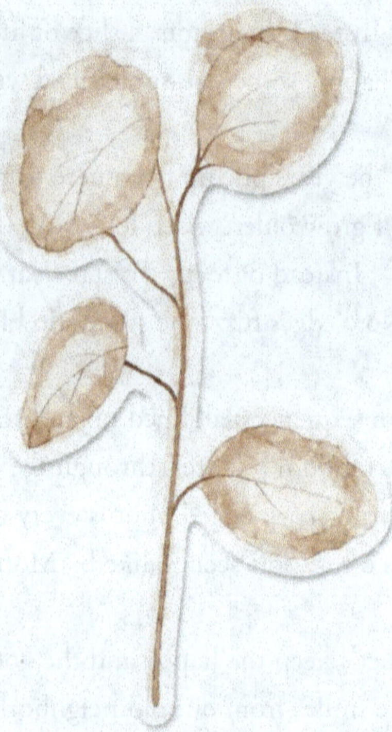

Tom: A Name

My name is Tom or Thomas.
That's what my folks called me.
A very good name, I promise.
It's who I choose to be.

Its history is Aramaic—
For a word that just means "twin".
Now that seems most archaic.
So where do I fit in?

For me it's been a family name—
Dates back five hundred years.
So, you must look far back to blame,
Your kinfolk, not your peers.

But Tom is me and me is Tom.
It's who I choose to be.
To change it would be like a bomb—
I might just have to flee.

And so, I thank my parents.
Those poor departed souls.
My name is a fine present.
It makes me feel quite whole.

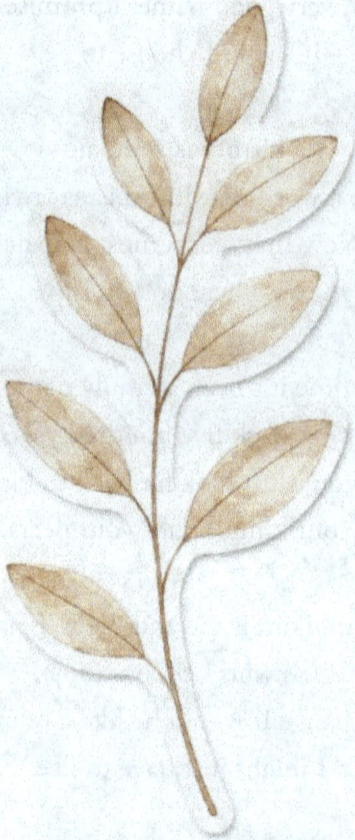

ReNew*

For us all on the road of life,
There are times that are easy, there are times of strife.
Times to run fast, times to fall down.
Did we get up, or did we drown?

For me, I fell hard in medical school.
'Twas freshman year, anatomy ruled.
The first test came; I dropped the ball.
Never studied before, how could I fall.
But fall I did, flat on my face.
Failed that first test—What a disgrace!

Support from others got me by.
Family, fiancée—they all did try.
They got me up, back on my feet.
Learned to study, enjoyed it—very sweet.
Did well, got honors, some success.
Hard lesson learned in life's game of chess.

*(Re=back or again) (New=not existing before)

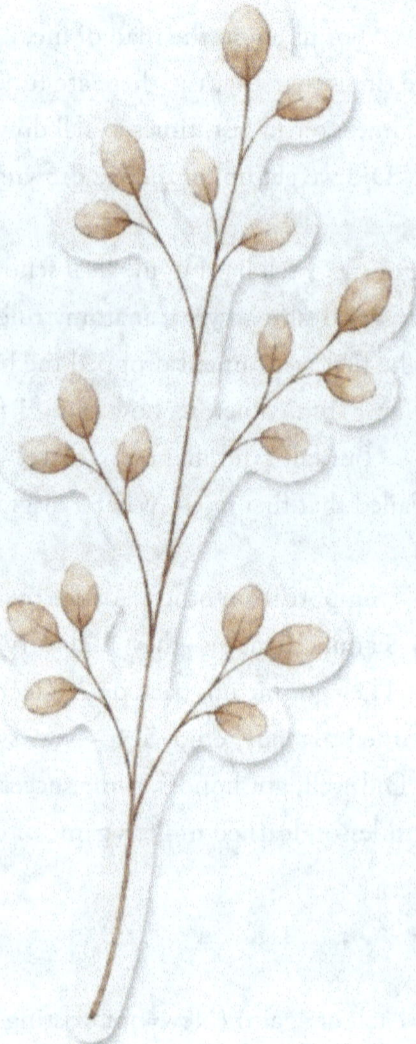

Discovering I Need Nature

As a med student in Texas, I'd sit at my desk—

People pressing, city pressing, it was truly grotesque.

Study hard, you'll find freedom, I said to myself,

But the workload just stared back from the nearby bookshelf.

On vacation some camping, or a trip to the ranch.

Gave me respite and solace—a sweet olive branch.

For in NATURE my spirits just soar like a bird.

In the cities, the walls squeeze—it is truly absurd.

So, I found out that for me there is an escape.

Leave the buildings, find some green space, and let peace just take shape.

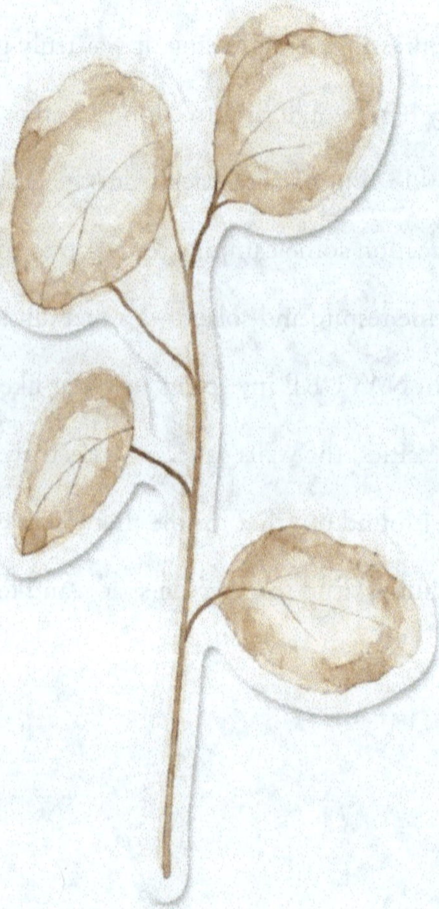

Orange

Orange is a color most unique.

Not black and dark, so very bleak,

Not white and clean, like new fall snow,

Nor hot and red, like ember glow.

Not deep, like purple, well revered.

No-- Orange is something slightly weird.

The color of pumpkins – Halloween.

Of falling leaves, that were once green,

Of Texas Longhorn football stars,

Of strangely painted antique cars.

A color of hair, that's not too sheik.

Yes, Orange is a color most unique.

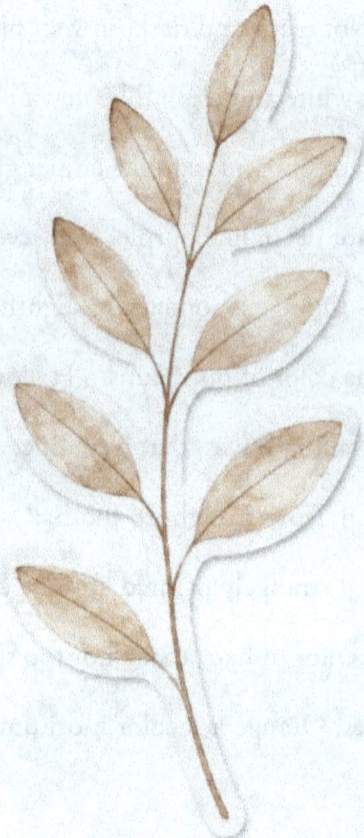

Haikus

Why write a Haiku?
Discipline applied to poems.
To prove that you can.

The sun is still out--
Yet days are getting shorter.
Summer's not done yet.

It rained yesterday.
Welcome relief to dry spell.
Plants are again green.

Swimming pool beckons.
Cool, blue, wet, and welcoming.
Now time to get wet.

Pandemic & Volunteering

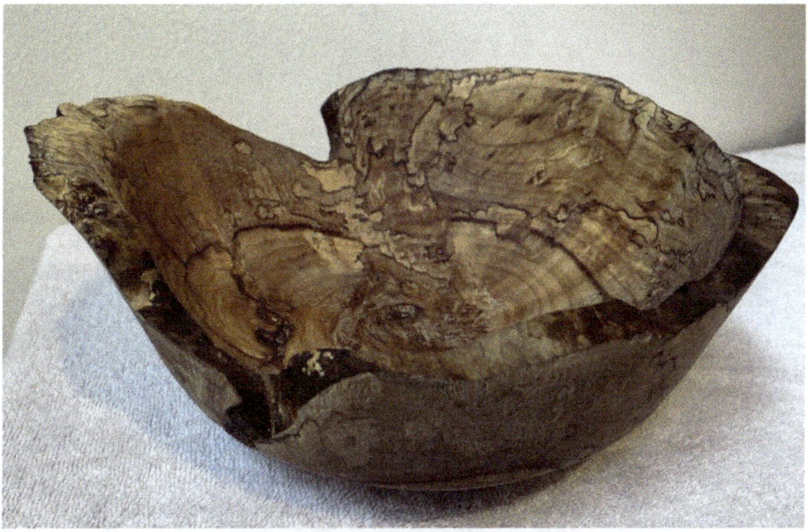

Natural Edge Spalted Maple Bowl

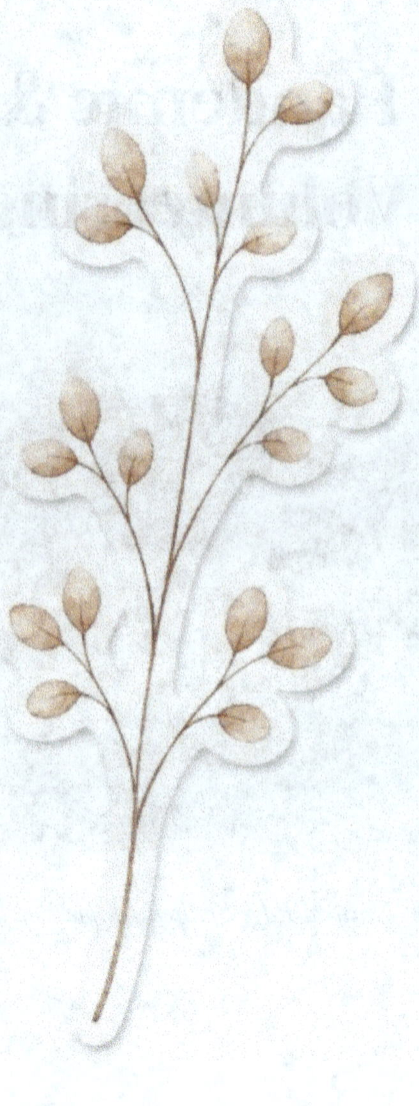

The Irony of Joy in a Pandemic

To find joy in the middle of a pandemic.
An exercise that's strangely academic.
And yet I find I'm feeling glad
For recent blessings I have had.

Good health for me and my family,
We've had through steps followed cannily.
Yes washing, yes masking, and distancing too.
We kept out Covid and even the flu.

But the biggest joy we've recently seen—
Came from a small jab of good vaccine.
The doors and windows opened a bit,
The path ahead more brightly lit.

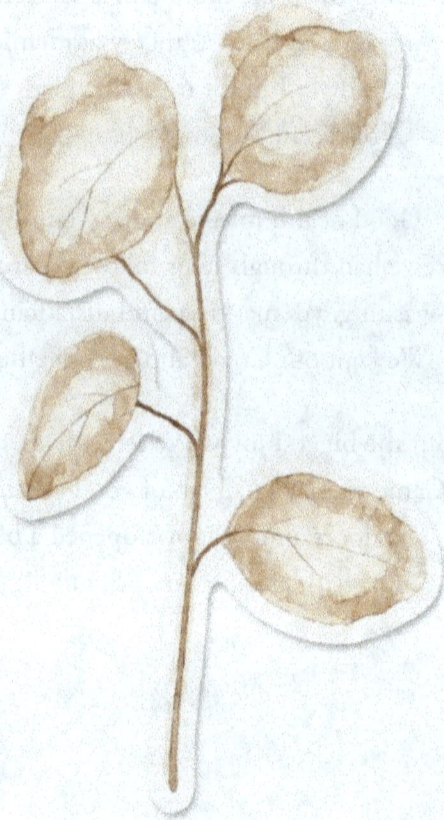

COVID: A Travel Companion

Early 2020—Sandy and I booked a tour to Ireland and Scotland—places where our families came from, but new destinations for us. COVID came in Spring 2020 with postponement of the tour to late 2020, early 2021, late 2021, and finally to May 2022. With worries about COVID Omicron in Europe, but equipped with vaccinations and travel insurance, we took off for Dublin.

It was a wonderful tour, except that we kept losing participants, including Sandy's brother, to COVID quarantine along the way. On the last day, we were required to have a negative COVID test prior to returning home to the US. Despite a lack of symptoms, Sandy and I both tested positive—this meant seven more days in the UK, or negative tests for both of us.

With vaccinations and no symptoms, the UK required masks and some social separation, but otherwise we were free to roam. What started with disappointment at not going home led to three wonderful and unexpected days in Edinburgh and four in London—all at the time of the Queen's Platinum Jubilee. We saw galleries, museums, parades, Edinburgh Castle, the Tower of London, and more. At seven days we both tested negative and were allowed to fly back to Seattle.

COVID, our travel companion, has proven, like many things, to be both a curse and a blessing.

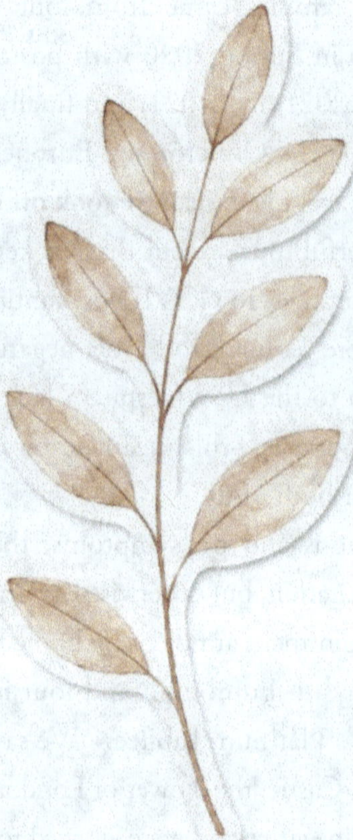

A Place to Belong

Can I see me, afloat in space?

No reference points, no sense of place.

Alone, just me, and nothing else.

Hard to imagine—only self.

That doesn't work, I cannot think,

Of myself only, at the brink.

We all fit in—words in our song.

A piece in place, we must belong, within a scene, not just a part.

We're not alone, it warms my heart.

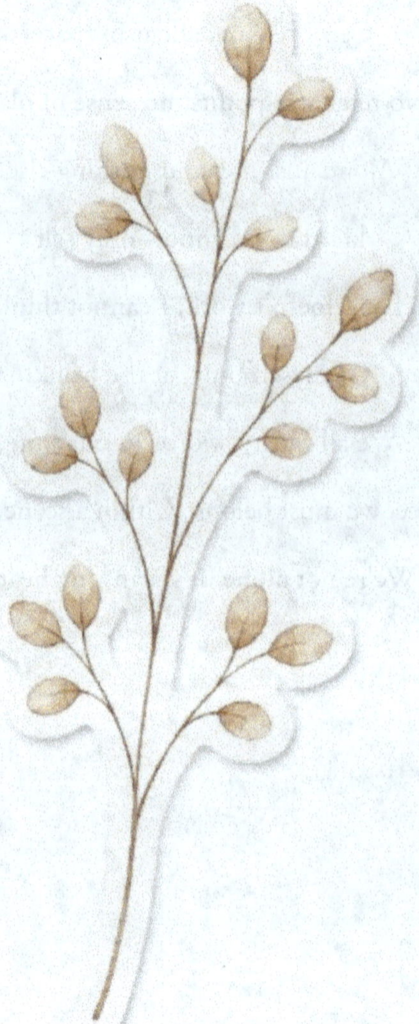

Thanks!

Considering things I'm thankful for,
The list is long, the numbers soar.
But in these days – retirement time,
The list is simpler – more sublime.

Retiring doctors face real change.
Busyness to slower – just feels strange.
From life that's filled with clear-cut purpose.
To leisure days, the shift usurps us.

One purpose-driven thing for me
Is volunteering time – you see.
One place that has become my haven,
Is a group of Docs that we call MAVEN.

It gives a chance to do some good,
For folks beyond our neighborhood.
It gives a way of "giving back",
So Old Docs don't get out of whack.

And as we near the next Thanksgiving,
Provides value to the life we're living.
So on my list – high in the ranks --
For MAVEN Project, I say "Thanks!"

Reflections on Aging*

Aging happens to all of us,
And with it change can happen too.
Change always happens—so what's the fuss?
It matters when it happens to you!
Some folks age and just lose touch.
Connections fade and purpose dies.
For trees and rivers—not so much.
They age but grow maintaining ties.

But what of us—old doctors all?
Talking was our job each day.
Purpose defined by helping all.
Will we fall quiet and lose our way?

Volunteering is an antidote.
To loneliness and loss of course.
We put it on like some great coat—
And feel a dose of NEW full force.

MAVEN is a tool I use.
Keeps connection and direction loss at bay.
Keeps colleagues linked, so I don't lose.
Touch with fellow travelers on the way.

It also gives some purpose goals.
Towards which I can safely steer.
Mentees and consults preserve my roles,
And keep my journey's focus clear.

So like the trees' and rivers' trip.
With added growth and strength through years.
I hope that time won't see me slip.
I journey on, but volunteer.

*Inspired by John Prine's "Hello in There"

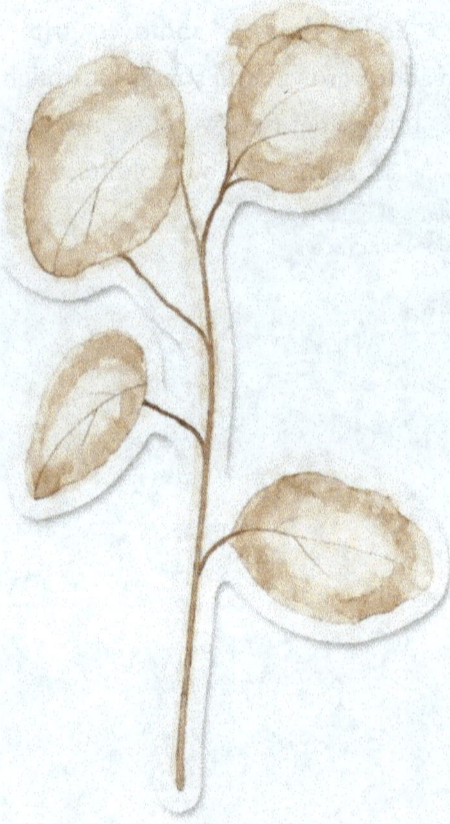

Be One with the World*

I say, "be one with the world."

Be not at anchor, with all sails furled.

Dig in, explore, live large, participate!

I say, "you matter", so don't delegate.

Don't sit and watch, a stone statue.

Soak up your life, let experience accrue.

I say meet people and be involved.

They are the answers, life's problems solved.

"Be one with the world"—I say to you.

It fulfills your life—I know that's true.

*Inspired by *Hokusai Says* by Robert Keys

Looking Deeper

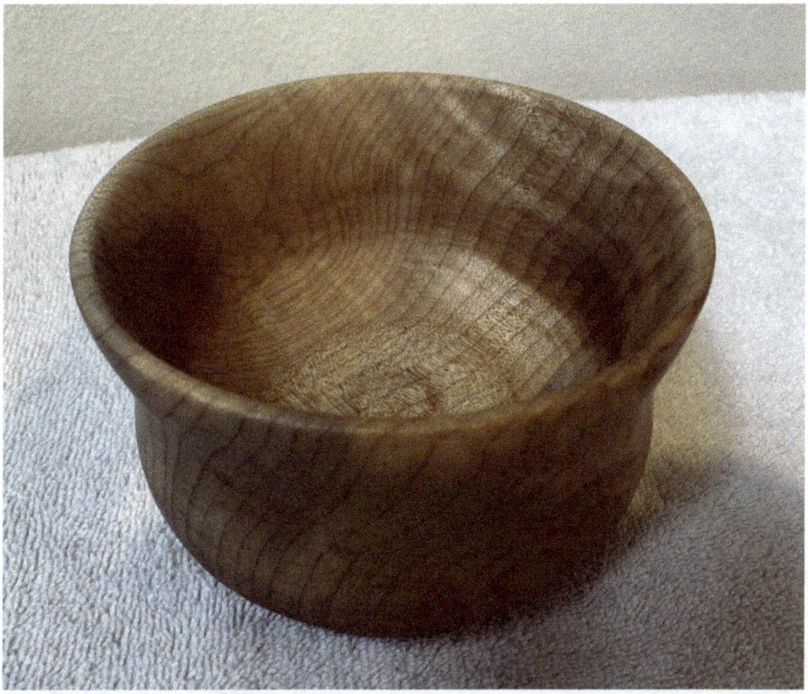

Maple Bowl

Tunnel Vision*

Concrete culverts laid on the ground—
Nancy Holt photo, quite renowned.
Meaning of this—left all to us.
To ponder, think, and then discuss.

Picture of pipes, we now look through.
Coming or going—which is
Future or past? Remains unknown.
Sad or happy? Group or alone?

The key is the pipe. Just look through.
Don't overthink or let thoughts skew.
Just a tunnel—a simple thing.
View through a tube; like a long ring.

See what is there and nothing more.
Not complex, twisted, without lore.
See just what is—escape the fluff.
For what is there should be enough.

*Inspired by *Sun Tunnels* photo by Nancy Holt.

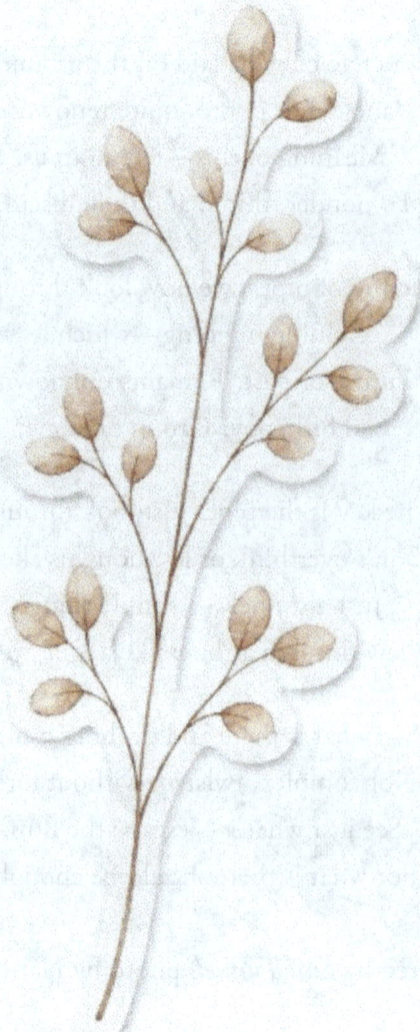

A Physical Hole or an Emotional Depression?

A hole can be a physical thing—
An opening, gap, or hollow.
It can also be a mental ding—
Too sad, too lonely, too dark to swallow.

But how to get out, when you've fallen in,
Or when neurotransmitters are just too thin?
In both cases don't cry or moan or yelp:
What you need, my friend, is someone to help!

For the physical hole, you need a rope,
A ladder, a push, or a helping hand.
For the emotional side, the answer's the same:
You just need someone to understand!

So be the one who helps the other.
Who's fallen in or just feels sad.
You can fix them both, right now you see—
And that, you'll find, is not so bad!

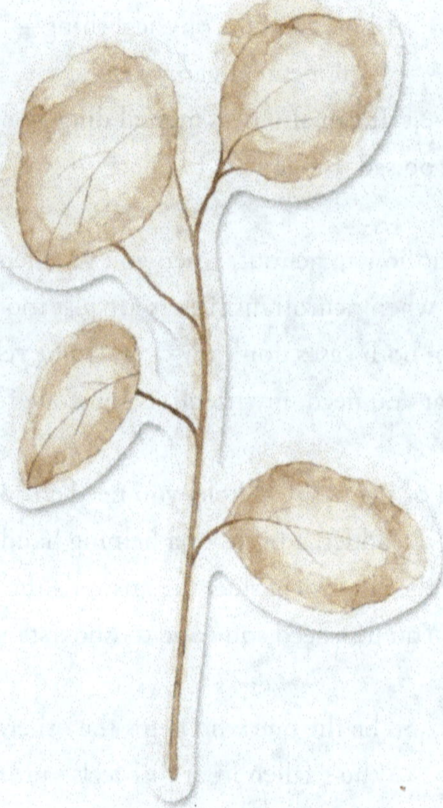

Inside the Chest*

Much is written about what is on the inside,
Of the chest in our bodies wherein we reside.

For doctors, like surgeons, we clearly see parts.
For cardiologists, functioning and hardworking hearts.

For poets and writers, the heart's not a pump.
It's the core of emotions, where our feelings clump.

For poets, the heart is an empathy vessel,
So active and useful with feelings to wrestle.

For writers the heart's the emotional core.
Authentic and vulnerable, passions do soar.

So what is seen depends on whose eyes do see,
Inside of the chest of people like me.

*Inspired by *Caring Enough to Look* sculpture by Lorri Acott

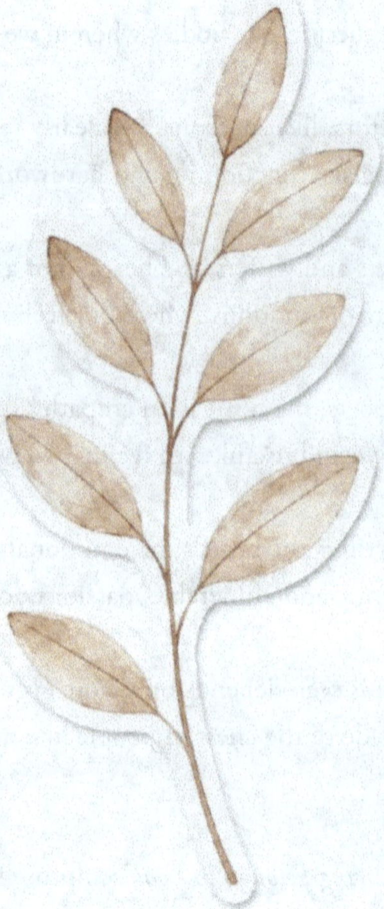

Beyond the Surface

As a doctor, I know I've committed the sin,
Oft engaged in by others, of my white-coat kin.
I've looked at a patient and seen only the surface.
Instead of listening and probing—providing true service.

So, what can we do to treat this disease?
Not the patient's, but ours—our guilt to appease.
The answer, I think, is to give more care and time.
If we do this, the results could be quite sublime.

But we live in a system where time's always pressed.
Hurry, hurry, go faster, the message is stressed.
So, we run faster, work harder, and miss more, no doubt.
While for many, this road is a trip to Burnout!

So, what is the answer? I fear I don't know.
As much as I want to, I cannot go slow.
Some help may come from sharing our concerns.
With others who do what we do—and so to learn.

The system needs fixing, no question of that.
But we each do too, or we will fall flat.
So, work with each other, my good white coat kin.
That's the best we can do for the mess that we're in.

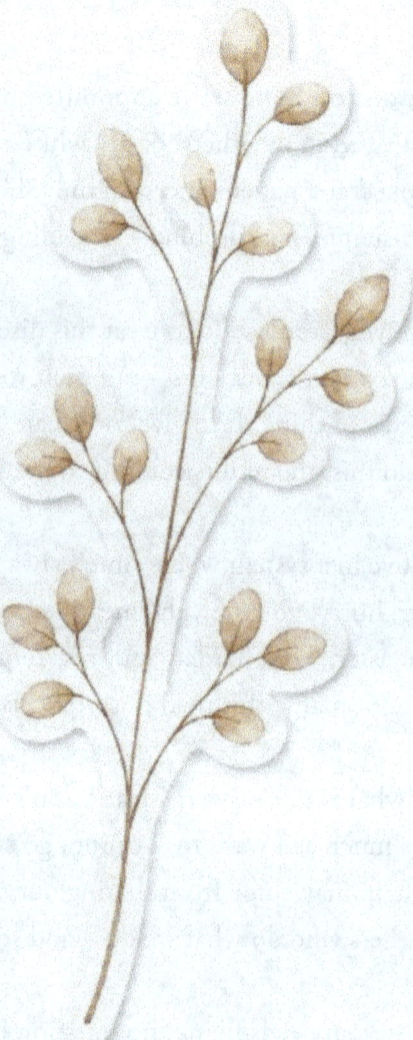

Helping a Dying Patient

Impending death, yet doctors as guides—
See one side only—the other hides.
Thinking they know and show empathy for,
But in truth, they see one side of the door.

And yet, our patients we try to calm.
Alay their fears, with emotional balm.
Do things all stop? Or do they extend?
Is another thing waiting around the bend?

We docs sound wise, like we know it all.
And patients take solace, while preparing their pall.
In truth, we do not know what hides—
Beyond the thick door—on the other side.

We wrap ourselves in science, get consultant's views.
As we struggle forward, with the patients we lose.
We do our best, that's all we can do.
When in truth, we really don't have a clue.

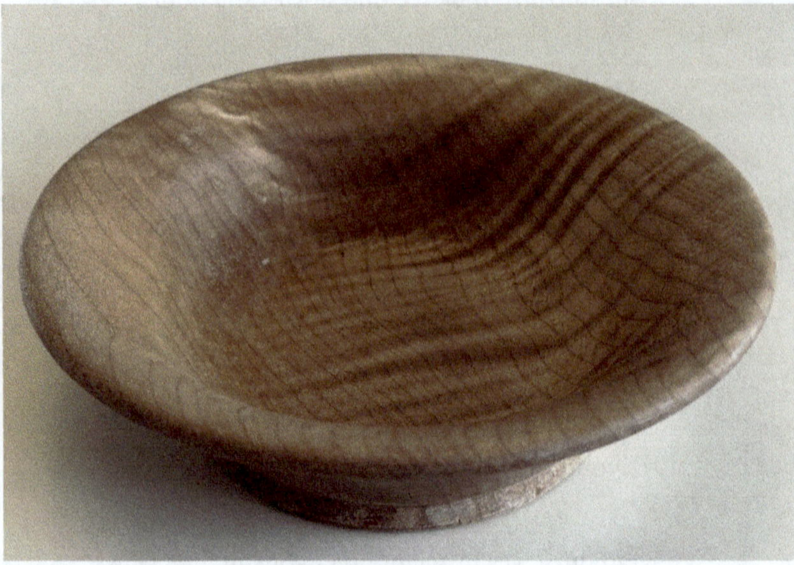

Filigreed Maple Bowl

Remembrance

On the Anniversary of 9/11/2001

Most memories flow like a very quiet stream—
Some ripples, but mostly a placid routine.
But sometimes a splash, like a high-jumping bream,
Engraves in our minds, a sharp vivid scene.

Most scenes fade to dust, not remembered at all,
But the splashes stick with you, d'you see?
They protrude from the rest, like a sudden rainsquall,
Or a tower that falls like a tree.

So how to sort out, what is important still,
As the years roll so rapidly by?
If the splash was for us, a really big deal,
Only time splits the joys from the cries!

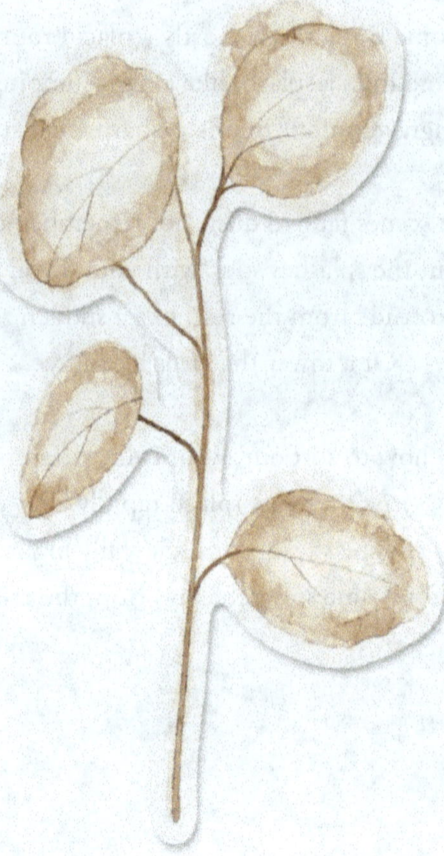

Choices*

As the road of life spreads out ahead,
As it has spread behind.
Choices we've made, with joy or dread,
Dictate the path we find.

For life is made of choices.
Of that there is no doubt.
The chorus of time's voices,
Some silent and some shout.

For Frost "The Road Not Taken",
Left questions in his mind.
For me each day awakened—
New answers there to find.

*Inspired by *The Road Not Taken* by Robert Frost.

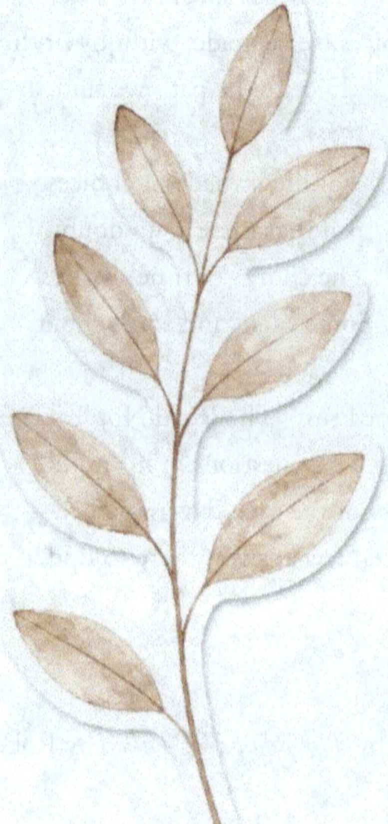

Thoughts on Renewal

Renewal is continuous—there is no clear beginning or end. Each day, each night offers the opportunity to begin again—to renew.

How do we do this?

Perhaps by looking at yesterday—What went well, what didn't? What should be included in the new version—

what should be left out?

Perhaps instead by looking at tomorrow. What do we hope to do, what do we hope to avoid?

Perhaps by simply impulsively diving into it. Letting the currents of our thoughts and the events of our lives take us where they may.

What's the best way? I'm not sure. Perhaps it's like a good recipe—a little of this and a little of that. Time will tell.

Life Journey

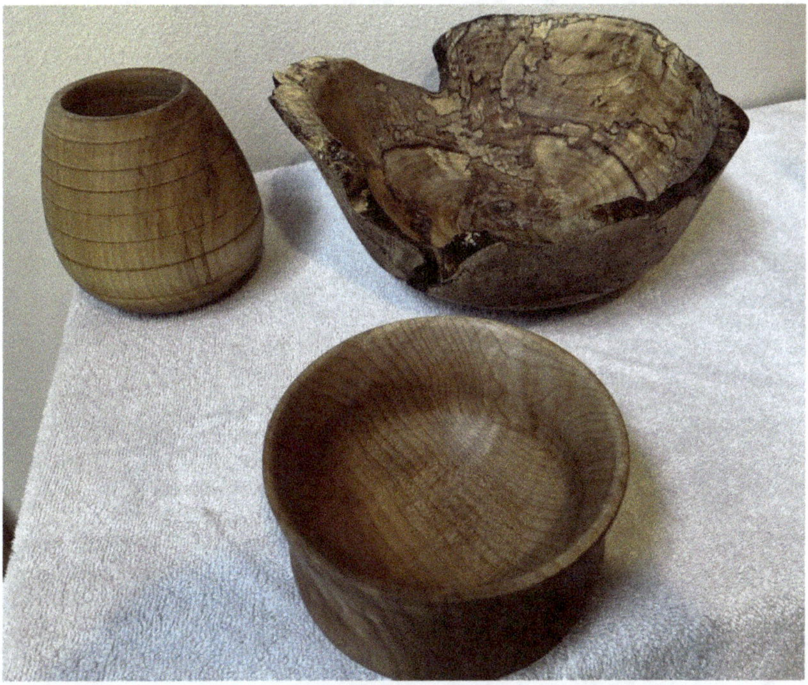

Three Maple Bowls

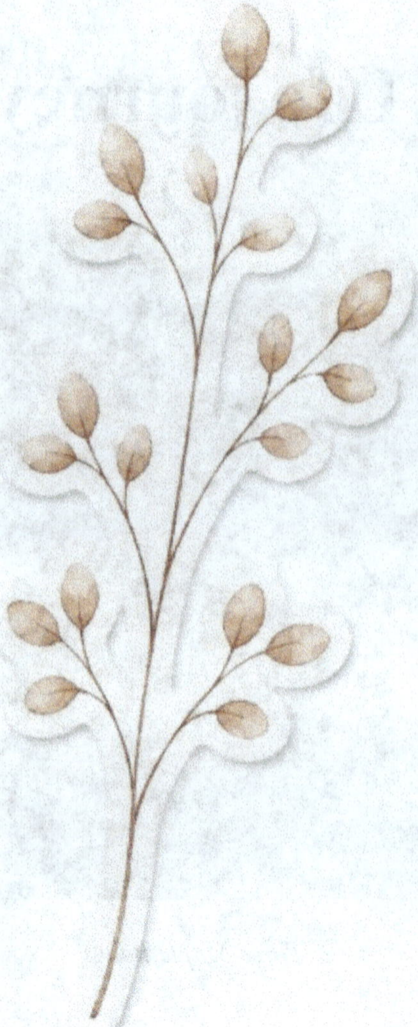

Sum of My Bookshelf

What fills the bookshelves of our minds?
Some things from parents, some from school.
Things from others our consciousness finds.
It mixes well and ferments--in our private mental pool.

Then what comes forth from this strange mix,
That all adds up to who we are?
Whether wisdom, fluff, or thoughtless bricks—
Are we normal or just bizarre?

I guess we're mostly pieces stirred—
Who knows from whence they come.
Some edges clear and some quite blurred.
They all add up to me—the sum.

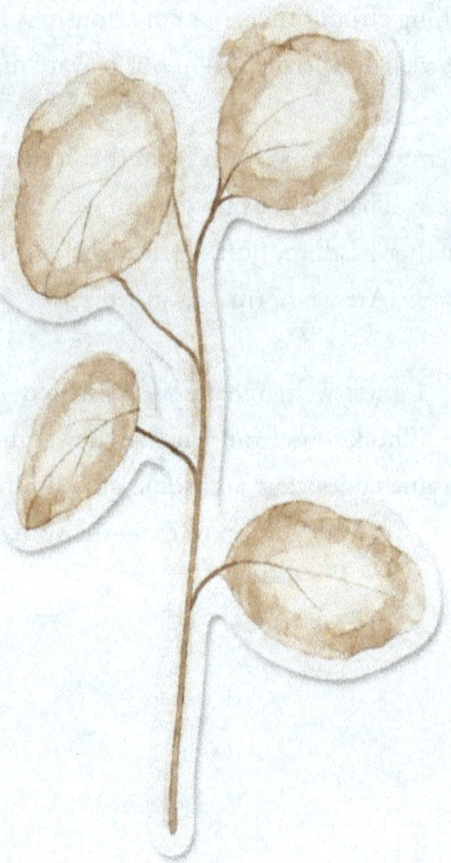

If I Could Only Share What I Know Now

Like Janus of the Roman age,
I look both back and 'fore.
I know that at the age I am,
More time is back than 'fore.

So looking back near eighty years,
What lessons have I learned?
Wish I could give my younger self,
Some ideas I've hard earned.

But time won't let me go back to,
The Tom of younger days.
I write my memoir aiming true,
At Grandkids' current phase.

Will lessons that I've learned help them,
Transcend the current mix,
Of polar views that are so dumb.
We're really in a fix.

I hope my musings help them out,
On their uncharted roads.
They'll make it through; I have no doubt.
They'll carry on our load.

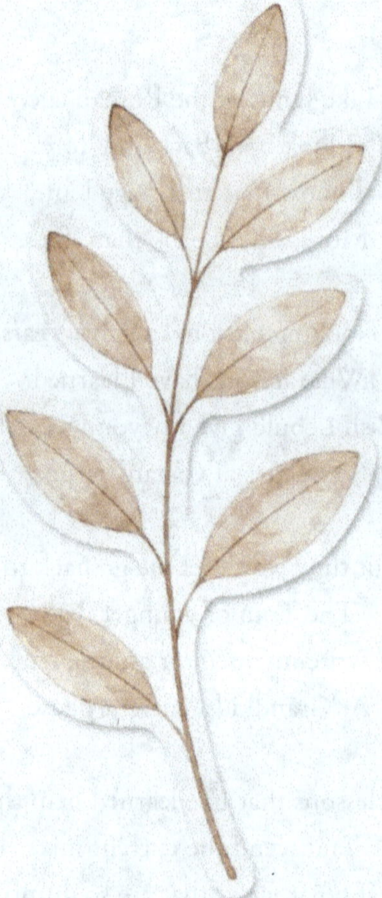

Thinking or Feeling

I'm not an emotional person.
I would rather think than just feel.
But this often can make my mood worsen.
Like an overripe peach, hard to peel.

So, I work to combine thoughts and feelings.
An integrated psyche—that's for me.
My hope that for me they'll be healing.
Less fractured and maybe more free.

I know that to feel is important.
Thoughts only, leave one incomplete.
I must keep me from being discordant.
Balanced life is most surely more sweet,

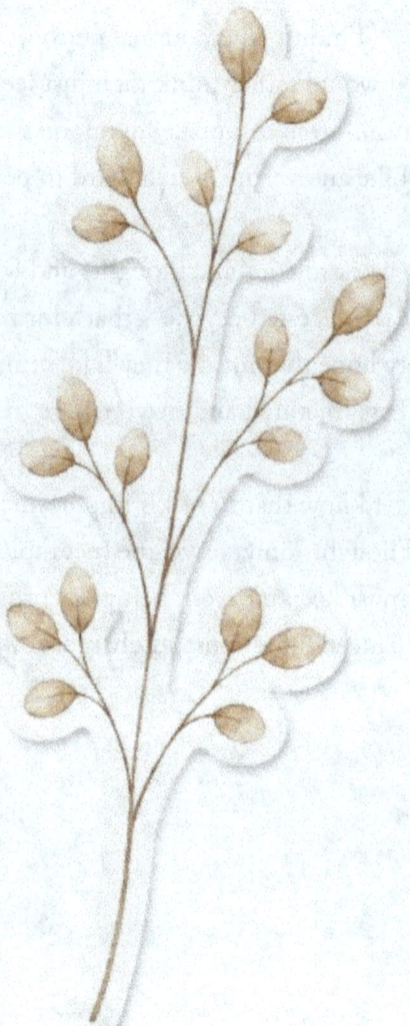

Thoughts on Unconditional Love

Love is not a trade good.
It's not for-give and for-get.
Instead, it's a feeling that is understood.
In life it's a real asset.

Love should be freely given.
No expectations allowed.
An emotion that's simply driven,
From your heart, as if speaking aloud.

So go out now and give love,
To someone you care about.
Expect no return to conceive of.
But happiness will certainly sprout!

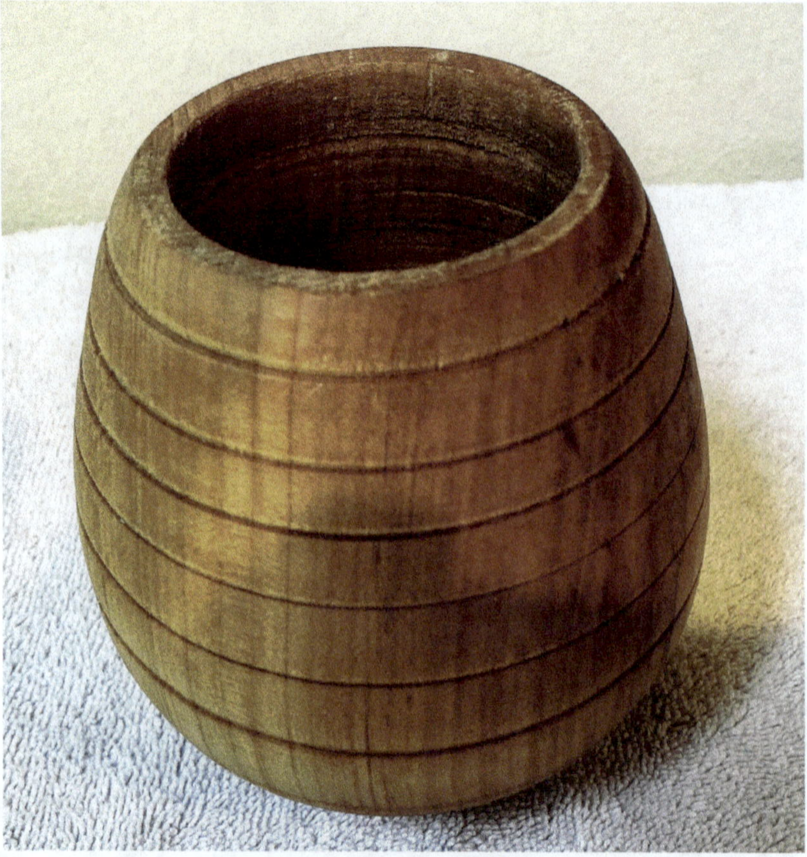

Grooved Maple Bowl

Querencia

Querencia's a word that's hard to rhyme,

But the concept is real, it's quite sublime.

Based on the Spanish verb, "to desire,"

But the idea is bigger—you must reach higher.

The thought describes a favorite place.

With fear and anger replaced by grace.

A place from which your strength does flow—

Into your mind to help you grow.

A nostalgic place of want and longing,

That makes you whole and gives you belonging.

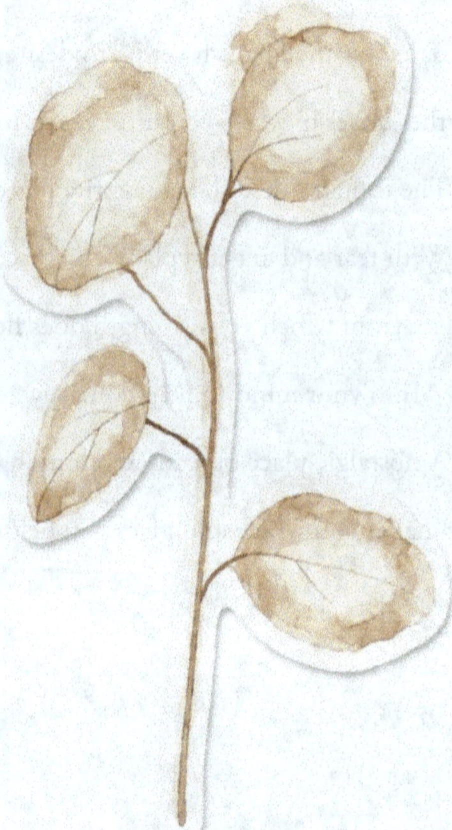

Time to Sell the Boat

Like a creature from the primordial swamp, salt water's in my veins.
From tiny tot to now old man, boats always in my brain.
Cape Cod sailing as a youth, bought first boat in medical school.
From small sailboats to big sailboats, to sports boat racing— every step was cool!
Recently motorboats, the trawler type, have been our happy place.
The Salish Sea has been our pond, with smiles on every face.
For all old sailors there's a time when age and health conspire.
Strength and agility fade away and it's now time to retire.
So, sell the boat, it is the time, although it makes me sad.
No plans for future vessel buys, no more for this granddad.
But it's not the end, for cruise ships sail, no need to sit and mope
We'll get back on the salty brine, and that will give me hope!

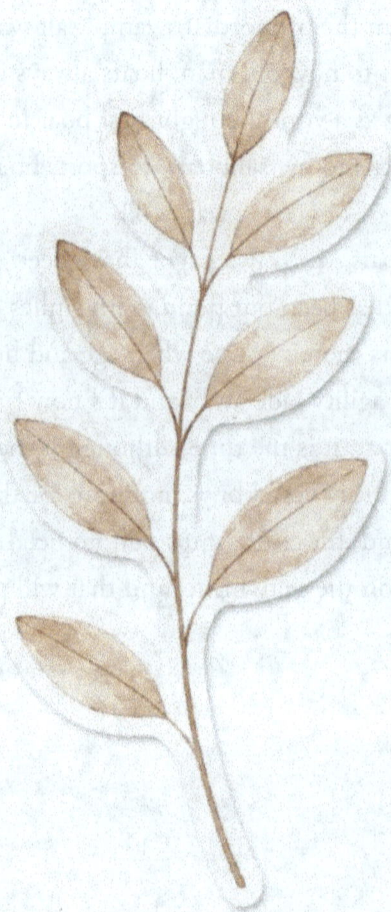

Just Like That!

Returning from a family trip—when things just seemed routine.
But fate can cause your plans to flip and change the whole big scene.

The physical scheduled months ago—the lab work just a part.
When I saw results, my heart beat slow. It must be the wrong chart!

But right it was, lab did not lie—I was sick but didn't know.
It hit me hard, bolt from the sky, this cancer won't move slow.

My disease was rare, prognosis bad, most treatment would not work
Stem cell transplant, only chance I had, it seemed a wicked quirk.

So "just like that" my future changed, it has been quite a year!
Now transplant's done, it was arranged, thank goodness I'm still here.

Thanks to science, family, friends and hope, it's working out all right.
I've learned to trust and even cope—ahead I see the light.

I'm back at MAVEN, mentoring on. Yes, giving back brings joy.
And like the sunrise after dawn, my old skills I employ.

For life needs purpose for success, whether feeling sick or well.
What happens next, it is a guess; That only time will tell.

Reflections on the End of Life*

If our last days end in a hospital bed,
With chaos all around.
Will those who are there show care for us,
Or will indifference be profound?

Will our end be like the mural above—
A complex horror show?
Or will we pass with dignity?
That's how I'd like to go.

I've spent my life as a small cog,
In the creaking health machine.
I've worked hard to make it better,
Yet I still hear the patient's scream.

But when it comes to my own end—
I'd like to die at home.
Or on the shore or nearby woods.
Places I love to roam.

For I don't trust the system—
That healthcare has become.
Good meds, machines, and people.
Can't drown its dull humdrum.

I hope to be surrounded,
With gentleness and care.
Avoid chaotic ICUs—
That often patient's scare.

Healthcare has a ways to go,
To reach that perfect goal.
Of care with dignity and peace
To ease a dying soul.

*Inspired by a mural ***73 cents*** by Regina Holliday

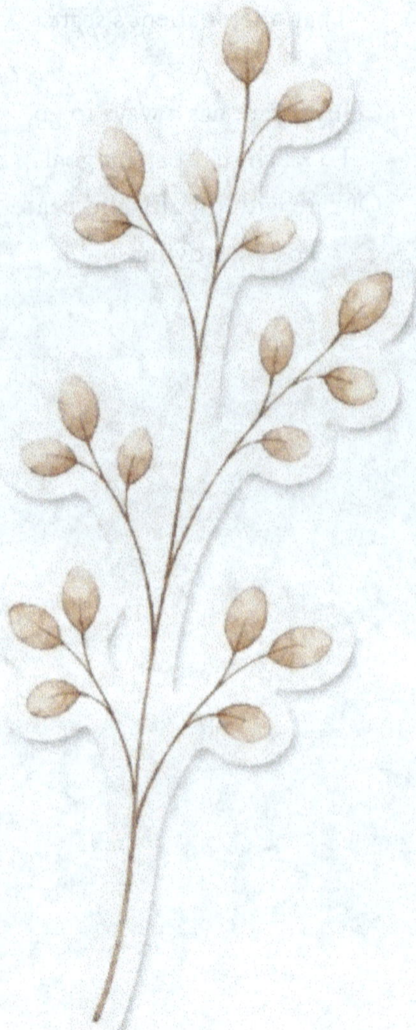

Hope*

So, what does hope still mean today,
In the autumn of my years?
In times now driven far astray—
By those who stoke our fears.

Emily* saw hope as a bird,
Found flying through a storm.
Although that idea is not absurd,
It does not keep me warm.

For hope I see a twinkling star,
Or a tunnel's ending light.
To me it's near and never far,
A hope-source shining bright.

My world must be a hopeful one.
The glass must be half full!
The future shining like the sun,
With me caught in its pull.

*Inspired by Emily Dickinson's *Hope is the Thing with Feathers*

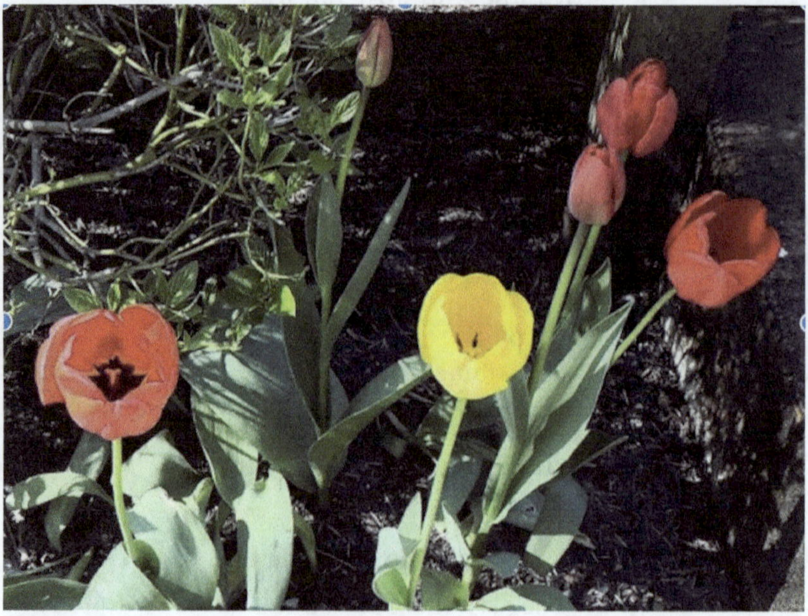

Skagit Tulips in Tom's Garden

Skagit Tulips

Like nature's perfect wineglass, the simple tulip stands.

All colors from the artist's wheel, this flower's never bland.

In Skagit Valley where I live, it is the mark of spring.

Farm fields streaked with celestial paint, as if the sky did fling.

Sparkling colors, sunny days, and winter's gone, oh boy.

Thank-full that a simple bloom can bring us so much joy!

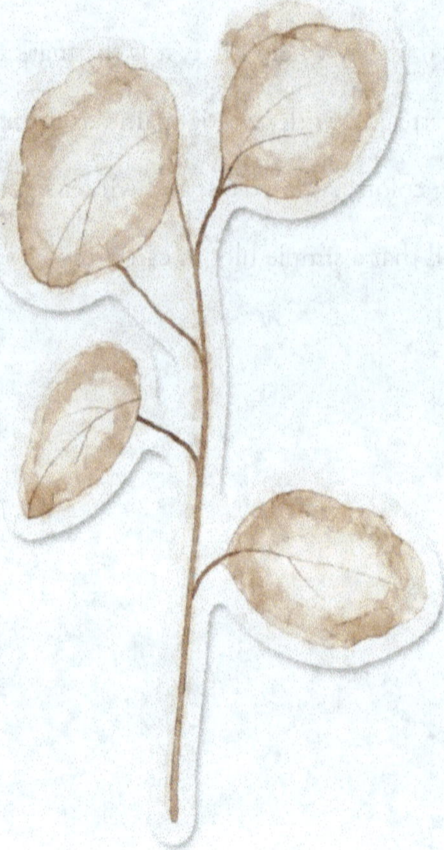

Hill

Life is like a mountain, or maybe a big hill.

You spend the first half climbing, and that can be a thrill.

You add knowledge, skills and networks— in-to your big backpack.

You manage things that come your way; you really have the knack.

Time at the top seems very short, the view does not last long.

So, savor every minute. These memories make you strong.

From there the trip is all downhill, the things you've gained get tossed.

It's hard to keep on smiling, it feels a lot like loss.

The rewards during the downhill walk are not in gold or glory.

Instead, they come from friends and fam who share your long hike's story.

For all that we leave behind us, when we finally leave this place.

Are in the love and memories of those whose lives you graced.

Epilogue

Capstone

If life were like a railroad track,
With future looking forward and past looking back,
Then as the years go sliding by,
The future years shrink and the past pile grows high.

As we each move along our life's railroad track,
Some beliefs or ideas we will place in our pack.
So these are the things that will guide our long trip,
And help keep us balanced and tighten our grip.

What are the ideas and beliefs that I've placed in my trunk?
I'll lay them out neatly, just like a slam dunk.
So here are these concepts, just one at a time
Like most of my writing, I do hope they rhyme:

- *Leave the world better than the place that I found,*
  Is as important to me as the world being round.

- *To keep family and friends at the top of my plan,*
  Without them you're nothing, we all need a clan.

- *To be good to others and always be kind,*
  Is one of my main stays, it eases my mind.

- *To live life with purpose and not waste my time,*
  A steep goal but important, keeps me in my prime.

- *To always be curious and using my brain,*
  I live in my thoughts, that is where I feel gain.

- *To be optimistic each day and radiate joy,*
  Making me and others happy is what I try to deploy.

- *To speak up, not shyly, and lead when I can,*
  For lack of direction, can hurt our lifespan.

- *To work hard, giving back only my best,*
  Has always been part of my personal quest.

- *To make good decisions, no matter the cost,*
  For taking life's shortcuts, results in great loss.

- *To pay close attention to fitness and health,*
  In the long term, worth much more than most kinds of wealth.

When we each reach the end of our personal track,
With no scenes looking forward, but great things looking back.
Heading out for our next stop, wherever it is,
Leaving only memories behind us, but this is no quiz.
What people remember is our legacy,
Keeps thoughts of us out there for eternity.

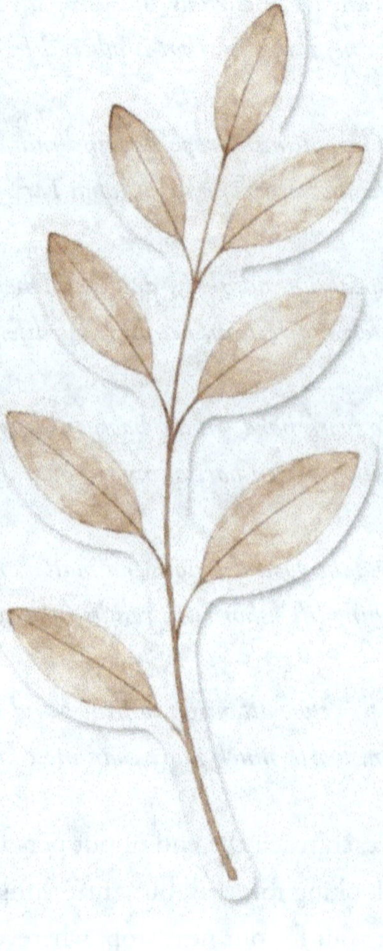

Acknowledgements

I thank MAVEN Project's leadership for sponsoring this book and the "Narrative and Humanity" writing group. The group has inspired creativity and built community among the physician volunteers who desire to tell and share their stories through writing and visual art, all making this book possible.

I am especially grateful to Dr. Jill Einstein, Senior Director of Physician Engagement, for her vision, ongoing involvement, and support in creating this book. Her commitment to MAVEN Project's mission and physician volunteer workforce has had a major impact on the success of the organization.

About the Author

Growing up in central Texas, the son of a college professor and community leader, I developed an early interest in science and service. The local general practitioners were my role models, leading me to decide at an early age that medicine would be my career.

Working on the family cattle ranch helped me understand the critical role of rural places and people, especially their need for healthcare. After college and medical school at the University of Texas Medical Branch, I did one of the early family medicine residencies at St. Joseph Hospital in Wichita, Kansas.

The Vietnam War was ongoing, and most of us had draft based military obligations after training. Thus, I spent two years in the 1970's as a Navy family doctor at the Naval Regional Medical Center in Long Beach, California. My next career stop was 10 years of full spectrum rural practice in a small town in central Montana. Having students and residents from the University of Washington's WWAMI program rotate through my clinic kindled a strong interest in teaching.

In 1988, I transitioned to academic practice, spending five years as Family Medicine Residency Program Director at Tacoma Family Medicine, followed by 23 years at the University of Washington (UW) School of Medicine in Seattle. At UW Medicine, I served in a variety of roles, including Vice Dean for Academic Affairs and Professor and Chair of the Department of Family Medicine. My entire academic career, as a teacher, clinician, and rural health researcher, kept me grounded and focused on what is important.

In addition to teaching students and residents, leading continuing medical education courses for the American Academy of Family Physicians was an annual activity for me. Having completed a Certificate in Medical Management at Tulane, with certification by the American Board of Medical Management and as a Certified Physician Executive, I taught medical management at the University of Washington School of Public Health.

Another chance to give back came through volunteer leadership roles in the Montana and Washington Academies of Family Practice, the American Board of Family Medicine, the American Board of Medical Specialties, and the Educational Commission for Foreign Medical Graduates.

Upon retirement from the University of Washington, I worked part-time for the Studer Group/Huron Consulting as a senior physician executive coach and speaker from 2016 to 2019. I am pleased to have received the John G. Walsh Award from the AAFP for lifetime accomplishments in family medicine leadership and the Marion Bishop Award from the Society of Teachers of Family Medicine for lifetime leadership and academic accomplishments in family medicine. Following Studer Group, I began volunteering for MAVEN Project.

I currently reside in Anacortes, Washington with Sandy, my high school sweetheart and life partner, we have three adult children, all involved in health care, and six grandchildren. Family is important. My hobbies include writing, woodworking, boating, and fishing.

Tom E. Norris, MD